THE COMPASS HEALTH TRANSFORMER

Your 72 Hour Blueprint
For Healthy Living.

by
Dr Chio Ugochukwu

Published by Compass International.
44546 Orchard Lane, Lancaster CA 93534

ISBN-13: 978-1475025187

Editing by Katie Corbett.

Printed in the United States of America.

Disclaimer and Terms of Use: The author and publisher have made every effort to ensure the accuracy and completeness of information contained in this book, we assume no responsibility for errors or omissions therein. No information contained in this book should be considered as physical, health-related, financial, tax, legal or medical advice. Your reliance upon information and content obtained by you at or through this publication is solely at your own risk. The author assumes no liability or responsibility for damage or injury to you, other persons, or property arising from any use of any product, information, idea, or instruction contained in the content provided to you through this book.

Dedication

This book is dedicated to my lovely wife, Ekene and to my children, Mmeli, Dili, Chiji, Mezu, Nnedi and all those trying everyday to live healthy lives.

Table of Contents

INTRODUCTION

The First step towards transforming yourself is learning as much as you can about yourself. This is why part of this book is dedicated to helping you do just that.

One of the reasons we never get round to taking care of our health is that we are too busy taking care of others.

This leads us to the problem of never having enough time. We wake up early to dash off to work and come back late at night. Sometimes we do not even have time for our spouses and kids.

At first glance, it might seem as if we have no time but a closer look reveals otherwise. Most of us have enough time to hang out with friends or watch our favorite game on TV.

If you have enough time to do any of these activities then you can spare 15 minutes to do your own health assessment. If you are not sure how to do this, this book will help you do that.

A Health assessment will give you an idea of where your are in your journey of health and healthy living. You might even be surprised by the things you will discover about yourself.

This is why the first part of this book talks about your, "getting to know yourself better." Of course, I do not cover every aspect of your health in this book. However, I discuss important topics like your risk for heart attacks and the influence of your weight on your overall health or well being. These topics as well as the findings from your initial

15-minute health assessment can be used as a foundation for developing your own blueprint for healthy living.

It is also important to recognize that the only way a blueprint for healthy living can work is if people believe they can change. Unless you believe you can change, a detailed explanation of how you can change will make no difference to your health.

Getting exactly the healthy lifestyle you desire will require setting realistic goals for yourself while sticking to a simple and easy to implement system.

The Compass Health Transformer is precisely such a simple system that is based on the Compass Health Profiles. In this book I explain what each profile means and how it is applied to your health.

Your 72 hour blueprint for healthy Living, will show you how to create an individualized healthy living blueprint that is developed over a 72- hour time frame but can be applied to your overall health in the long haul.

The blue print given in this book can be easily modified to suit your own needs and circumstances. The most important thing you need to do for healthy living is to stick to a simple plan that fits your lifestyle, while ignoring daily distractions.

PART I

GET

TO KNOW

YOURSELF

BETTER

Find Out Your Health Status

Assess your health. Find out how healthy you are and the potential problems you may have in the future and how you can prevent or modify them.

Some people try to find out about their health by their feelings. If they feel good about themselves then they consider themselves healthy. Others look in the mirror and if they like what they see, they give themselves a passing mark.

Although this approach to finding out one's health status is not accurate, some people like to use this approach because it helps them avoid asking the hard questions about their health.

The problem with these two methods of assessing one's health is that they are very subjective. They both depend only on your opinions of yourself based on what you see and what you do not see, but not based on what others can easily verify or quantify.

Let's face it! Most of us think we are very healthy. This is a common thought for young adults and those in middle age.

Yet we all know that looks can be deceiving. I am sure you have all heard stories of people who were apparently very healthy then suddenly died from a heart attack or after a "brief illness."

One way to take a more objective assessment of your health is to start by taking simple measurements of your physical and physiological attributes by yourself. Find out your weight and your height and using both figures with your age calculate your body mass index (BMI). Why is your BMI important? It helps you to find out your likelihood of having heart disease, diabetes or some cancers.

Wow! Wouldn't you like to know the risk for such deadly killers? You can even take your health assessment one step further by finding out what your blood pressure is. If you have a blood pressure cuff, measure your blood pressure today. If you do not have one, go to the nearest pharmacy store, and use their free blood pressure cuff to find out your blood pressure.

The steps outlined so far are things you can do for yourself now, especially if you feel you are healthy but have not taken any objective steps to check your health in years. Maybe your last health check was in school.

For an even more detailed health assessment visit your primary care provider for a physical. This will not only help you know your weight, but you can also get your blood work done to find your cholesterol level and other relevant tests based on your age, family and medical history.

Getting this kind of detailed blood work will enable you to even assess your risk for more serious health concerns like breast, prostrate, lung and colon cancers as well as heart disease. The best way to check for these common cancers is through regular physical examination and recommended screening tests for your age group.

TASK OF THE MOMENT.

*Take action today.

*Find out about your family medical history.

*Weigh yourself today.

*Measure your blood pressure today.

*Measure your BMI today.

*If you are having difficulty calculating your BMI, visit compasswellnessinstiute.com and do it there.

Know Your Cardiovascular Risk Factors And How You Can Modify Them

It is very important that any adult who is interested in living a healthy life learns how to assess his or her cardiovascular risk factors and how to modify those that can be modified. Would you not like to know what is your probability or chances of having a heart attack in the next 10 years?

Yes, I would because heart disease is among the leading cause of death for middle-age men and women in most parts of the world, including the United States and Western Europe. Even in developing countries like Nigeria the trend toward more deaths related to heart disease is becoming more common.

This is why finding out the risk you have for diseases or health conditions that are common to both where you live, age or gender is an important part of healthy living. A common cause of problems for people starting in their thirties is a stroke or a heart attack.

The problem is that most of us still feel that heart attacks are things that happen to others. We do not feel it will happen to us, so we take little or no precautions to modify our risks for such adverse health events.

Factors that are used to calculate your cardiovascular risk factor include:

*Age

*Sex

*Race

*Family history of heart disease or diabetes

*Lipid profile as stated above.

*BMI

*Personality type

Age, sex and race are factors that cannot usually be changed, but you can use them to calculate your cardiovascular risk points and then convert the points to percentage risk for heart attack over a 10-year period.

Knowing your lipid profile is important because you can use it in computing your cardiovascular risk. Your lipid profile, includes, your triglyceride level, total cholesterol, HDL(High Density Lipoprotein) or good cholesterol, and LDL (Low density Lipoprotein) or bad cholesterol.

Here is an example of the cardiovascular points for a 45-year-old- man Joseph with a low HDL (<35) and a total cholesterol of 220 and a blood pressure of 130/80 mmHg, who is not diabetic but smokes. Being a 45 year old male, would give him 6 points, If he was a woman the points would be 5. A HDL of less than 35 would give him 2 points. Total cholesterol of 220 would be equivalent to 2 points. Smoking would give him 4 points, while a blood pressure of 130/80mmHg is equivalent to 3 points.

This calculation means Joseph has (6+2+2+4+3)=17 points and would translate to at least 29.4% risk of cardiovascular disease(CVD) in 10 years .What does this mean?

According to the Framingham Heart Study, moderate risk ,is a 10 year CVD risk of less than 10%,moderately high risk is 10-20% and high risk is 20%and above. This means that Joseph has a high risk for cardiovascular disease. For Joseph, the man in this example, his numbers mean that 29 out of 100 people with his risk profile will have a heart attack in the next 10 years This is too high a risk as confirmed by the Framingham Heart Study.

The advantage of finding out your risk factor before having a heart attack is that it gives you an opportunity to take action. For, Joseph he can change his risk for a heart disease by quitting smoking, this will take away,4 points from his 17. Making his HDL 50 and his total cholesterol less than 160, would give him points of (-1),and (0).This means his new total CVD points will be (6+(-1)+0+0+3)=8, which will be equivalent to 6.7%,10 year risk of CVD.

Essentially this means that by taking action and modifying his risk factors through eating more healthy and quitting smoking, Joseph reduced his risk of having a heart attack by more than half. He changed his risk of a heart attack from 29 out of 100 people in 10 years to 7 out of 100 people in 10 years, for people with a similar heart risk profile.

Wow! I hope you are as excited as I am; with just a few changes to our eating habits and lifestyle changes we can minimize our risk for a life threatening event like a heart attack. Do these numbers and percentages look confusing?

Do not worry, it is not that confusing. You can calculate your own personal risk of having a heart attack by visiting http://hp2010.nhlbihin.net/atpiii/calculator.asp

I am certainly looking forward to sharing more simple and fast ways you can develop a blueprint that will help you transform your health. One of the foundations of such a blueprint is dependent on your applying your compass health profiles to your health. Taking such a step will help you to modify not only your cardiovascular risk factors but other risk factors to your health.

TASK OF THE MOMENT

*Find out your cardiovascular risk factor today.

*Find out your family medical history.

How To Use The Compass Health Profiles To Transform Your Health

In case you have forgotten the compass health profiles which is the foundation for my health compass pathway for healthy living, I will list them here once more.

The Compass Health Profiles:

C = Community Relationships.

O = Operational capacity profile.

M= Metabolic profile.

P= Physical profile.

A= Ambition profile.

S= Spiritual profile.

S = Self Knowledge profile.

How do you use these profiles to help you live a healthier and happier life? According to current medical research those who have good **community relationships** with themselves, their family and their friends tend to live longer and healthier lives.

When was the last time you said, "I love you" to your spouse or lover? When was the last time you called your brother or sister? When was the last time you forgave yourself? When was the last time you shared a joke with your co-worker? What if you are from a dysfunctional family? What if you are not even on talking terms with your brothers and sisters? Don't sweat it. Just make a phone call or send a text message.

Answering these questions will help you recognize your own relationship stress triggers. It will help you understand yourself better and become a better manager of the conflict that inevitably occurs within different types of relationships. Just remember that you can also make your friends part of your family. After all, good companionship from those we live with and interact with everyday helps us live longer and better.

I don't really want to make things more complicated than they need to be. Basically through your **operational capacity profile,** you ask yourself how you get things done and how you can improve. The simplest way to do this is to look back at your life and find out which method of preparation and execution has worked the best for you in your most successful projects.

Include in your projects things like getting ready for Christmas and Thanksgiving or getting ready for a wedding or tasks as simple as going to work on time and cleaning your house. For most people, the best way to tackle most projects is to start on time and break them down into small simple steps. For others every project is eventually done at the last minute.

If you like to get things done at the last minute, it means you tend to procrastinate and underestimate how much time you need to get things to done. This is a recipe for stress unless you learn to start doing things early like my father in-law "Ogene" who always did things on time. His favorite saying was, "Start early, finish early, and reduce stress."

Your **Metabolic profile** will include both your nutritional and metabolic analysis. You get your metabolic analysis by getting your physiological and laboratory tests done. This will include your blood pressure, cholesterol level and other metabolic tests your doctor deems necessary. Of course getting these results will make it easy for you to know which aspect of your health profile you need to focus on improving. This was precisely what happened to my friend, Philip, who thought he had excellent health until a pharmacy blood pressure checkup showed his blood pressure was 160 mmHg over 110 mmHg. Needless to say, the result startled him and he went to see his doctor the very next day. This is what I call putting your metabolic profile to good use. Do you know your Metabolic Profile?

I am not going to say much more about your **Physical Profile** which includes your weight, height and BMI. I have already talked about it in the chapter on health assessment.

The Ambition profile looks at your job and finances and satisfaction with your life. This is important because without good finances or insurance it is much more difficult to take good care of your health. I know most health books do not include this profile but the Ambition profile measures your ability to live a healthy life. Think about how you feel when you go to fill a prescription and you do not have the money to make the payment or the insurance that covers it.

The remaining two profiles are **Spirituality and Self Knowledge**, both of which examine your psychospiritual makeup. They will help you have a better understanding of your personality, character and connection with God and the universe. A better understanding of your psychological strengths and weaknesses will help you know your limitations, when it comes to choosing pathways to better health. On the spiritual side of the equation, more and more studies are beginning to show that those who meditate or are truly prayerful are better able to handle health challenges than those who do neither.

If you want even more detailed analysis of the uses of the different Compass Health Profiles, visit www.compasswellnessinstitute.com.

TASK OF THE MOMENT

*Begin to work on one Compass Health Profile today.

*Start with the Physical profile if you need to increase your level of physical activity.

* Go for a walk today.

*Work on your Metabolic and Community Relationship Profiles daily.

*Eat at least one apple per meal.

*Say something nice to someone today.

*Call someone who has hurt you the most.

*Forgive yourself and others frequently.

*Meditate today.

Set Realistic Goals For Yourself

Learn about your health and what you should do. First, do a health assessment to get an idea of your physical status or health condition. Next go to your physician to obtain a complete physical exam. This will put you in a position to set realistic goals for yourself.

In setting goals for yourself, incorporate the seven compass health profiles into your understanding of yourself and your achievable goals. Otherwise, setting the wrong goals will lead to failure and disappointment.

Do not let the absence of a full physical examination hinder you from setting goals for yourself. For example, if your BMI shows that you are overweight, you already know you need to make losing weight part of your individual health goal. Then start exercising as part of your goals. You do not need to wait till you see your doctor before you start engaging more in activities that will help you lose weight.

Remember that the journey of a thousand miles begins with one step. You do not have to wait until you join a gym before you can decide to start exercising or finding ways to increase your weekly physical activity. You can start to change your health now by taking action today.

Part of your goal setting will include identifying your risk factors for common diseases for your sex and your age group as well as risk factors peculiar to your family. We all know that some diseases occur only in males or females while some other illnesses like alcoholism, glaucoma and hypertension may be associated with strong family histories. This is why I started this book by discussing your health assessment and health profile.

If you have a family history of high blood pressure then start monitoring your blood pressure by checking your blood pressure every month. You can do this by buying your own blood pressure cuff or simply getting a reading of your blood pressure from your grocery store or pharmacy. It will not cost you a cent.

Doing your initial health assessment and gaining understanding of yourself through the Compass Health Profiles can help you create an individualized health plan. This book will show you some ways you can use the Compass Health Transformer to make your journey to healthy living easier and more effective.

TASK OF THE MOMENT

*Set one goal for yourself today.

*Take action to achieve your goal without excuses.

*Write down your goal and the time and activities you will need to achieve it.

*Break up your goals into small easy to achieve components.

*Keep your activities and daily tasks to about 30 minutes a day every week.

*Walk 30 minutes a day at home, at work or during recreation or shopping, everyday for one month.

*Have a remedy for your potential relapses.

Believe You Can Change

One of the saddest things that I have seen happen to people after they have taken their time to do their health assessment and set goals is that they still doubt if they can really change.

They find a thousand and one reasons why, making small but consistent lifestyle changes will not lead to a happy and healthy life. Sometimes this notion comes from looking at the past or thinking of past attempts at either losing weight or trying to get healthy.

At other times, the fear that one cannot change comes from trying to do too much at a time. In this situation people try to change everything at once. I tell them it is like trying to make your first marathon at the Boston marathon without any prior training or preparation. This kind of approach will lead to failure and discouragement.

After your initial health status, instead of worrying about big changes or worrying about consistency in small steps, choose the action that fits into your schedule and circumstances at that moment in time.

This was precisely what my friend, Jose, did. After finding out from his initial health assessment that he was overweight, he decided to start walking one block a day. He would wake up early in the morning, dress and get out of the house. Victory number one. He had made it to the street. Next, he would aim to walk to the nearest electric pole in his street. From one pole to another and before he knew it, he walked his first block ever.

Jose had never done any exercise in his life. Forty years old and he always believed he would not be able to do all that 'stuff.' After his first walk round the block in his neighborhood, he was convinced beyond doubt that he could change because he had his first victory ingrained in his mind.

I truly believe anyone can improve their health by using any number of the ways to good health that I outline in this book. Most people know they can change, but lack that conviction or motivation to begin their journey of healthy living.

Once motivated, you can take your first simple step to get back to good health. In one example, one young man who weighed 400 pounds and was on his third visit to the emergency room in one week was motivated to change when his emergency room physician told him he was going to die before the end of the year. The look of terror he saw in his son's eyes was the final straw. The next day he took his dog for a walk and continued walking his dog without fail, come rain or sunshine. He lost 100 pounds in six months. He attributes all his success to his first walk with his dog which he calls his "first victory."

Get your first victory. Your first victory might not come from walking the dog, like the 400-pound young man. It might come from switching white bread to wheat bread or from saying "No" to candies or soda. Whatever it may be just "get your first victory." The subsequent change in your mindset will trigger "will power" to carry you through the period of change.

TASK OF THE MOMENT.

Get yourself motivated.

Get your "First Victory."

Take a simple action today.

Give up soda.

How To Get Exactly The Healthy Life You Desire

Realize that you are responsible for your health. Start practicing the ways to live the healthy life that you desire.

My hope in writing this book or my sharing the Compass Health Transformer System for healthy living was to help awaken people. When you are healthy, you will find yourself more energetic, more tolerant and even more able to enjoy life.

Living healthy, happy lives requires a lot of discipline and responsibility. It requires finally deciding on what you want out of life and having a plan to do it, despite your doubts and fears. I know you can do it.

Most people want to live healthy lives, but they fail because they don't decide to stick to a plan. They get caught up in trying different complicated diets; and as soon as a lapse occurs in the diet requirements, they promptly drop a plan and start another one.

This action is like someone who wants to fly to New York from Los Angeles and who misses his flight and is told by the airline to wait as a standby, passenger for the next flight. The person then decides that he would take whatever was boarding and then make connections to New York from there even if it was going to Hawaii, since he did not like waiting.

Do not laugh at him, because this is the type of thing we do when we run out of fruits and vegetables and decide to snack with candies and cookies to make up for it. After all, we reason, we had to eat! I call it-"the-missing-your-flight-plan." Sometimes this stems from not trusting the plan; other times it stems from being indecisive. According to Karin White, "Indecision is the enemy of success."

If you decide on what you want and believe it, other opportunities will open for you. If you agree to follow the simple outline I share with you in this book, you will succeed in living a healthy, happy and fulfilled life.

Of course, simply wanting to be healthy is not enough. Even choosing a given outline or plan of action is not enough unless you actually act. Once you have made up your mind up which approach to healthy living is best for you, you need to follow through by taking daily steps on the road to success.

TASK OF THE MOMENT.

*Do not add salt to your meals.

*Start an easy to do physical activity, like gardening, walking or swimming to help you lose weight immediately.

*Take consistent daily action starting from today.

*Do not eat more than six slices of bread per day.

*Measure your blood pressure daily.

PART 2

CREATE

YOUR OWN

INDIVIDUALIZED

72 HOUR BLUE PRINT

FOR HEALTHY LIVING.

Define Your Own Idea About The Meaning of Successful Living

Determining what we mean by successful living is a crucial step in creating your own blueprint for healthy living. Having a clear idea of what your destination looks like will help you know when you get there. Take a pen and paper and write down your own definition of the meaning of successful living.

Generally in society success is judged by what you do for a living like your profession; how much money you have or where you live. You are considered unsuccessful if you are assessed not to have the right type of any of these categories. This view or approach misses the point. Successful living is more than attributes of success. Some people acquire professional titles and wealth and still find themselves unhappy.

Success is the ability to deal with the challenges of daily living on your own terms while living in love with yourself and others. An anonymous author defined it as the ability to find some sense of personal fulfillment in circumstances where others can only see madness.

Nelson Mandela found personal fulfillment even when he was imprisoned for his principled stand against apartheid in South Africa. Even if we find ourselves falsely accused through trumped-up charges, we can still succeed by holding on to our dignity and realizing that we can still make our own destiny.

Terry Fox, the Canadian cancer amputee who ran a marathon across Canada on one leg is an example of successful living. He did not let the devastating diagnosis of cancer of the leg stop him or make him bitter. Instead, he turned his cancer and amputation into an inspiration for one nation and the world. His courage and determination spoke volumes.

He was another example of someone making their own destiny. In other words, while we cannot choose the cards life deals to us, we can always determine how we will react to the cards we have been dealt.

We cannot live happily or successfully if we spend our whole time complaining about how things are or how things should be. If we find ourselves in circumstances we do not like, we should find a way to make it right. The first step towards doing this is to know yourself better by gaining a deeper understanding of your sense of self. Psychologists call it the "I" in you. What is your vision of yourself?

Sometimes it is easy to find yourself at other times we have to go through a complicated series of life lessons, that may involve mistakes and consequences.

These lessons will help us set up our own healthy living goals, with plans that specifically suit our sense of self. Once you find yourself everything becomes easier because you become much more self- confident. Your goals, aspirations and plans for achieving them become clearer and more attainable.

The key to successful living is self knowledge and self confidence. Being confident is not easy. It may require dealing with negative comments that people make about you. Be truthful to yourself and accept valid criticism without losing your focus. Stick to a plan that suits your understanding of your personality and spirituality.

TASK OF THE MOMENT.

*Know yourself and your own boundaries.

*Do not allow others to define you.

*Resist the urge to want to please others.

* Write your own summary of your strengths and weaknesses.

*Always seek to improve.

*Take daily success steps.

*Do not be discouraged by failure.

*Write down what success means to you.

Never Give Up On Yourself And Your Healthy Living Goals

Never give up on your healthy living goals, no matter your results. Do not give up on yourself. Become flexible without getting discouraged. If for example you planned to lose 20 pounds in two months and you find out, you have only lost 15 pounds, what will you do? Will you quit or give up on yourself?

First, find out what you were able to do so consistently that helped you to lose the 15 pounds that you have lost so far. This is your hook. It is what works for you. Keep it up. If you do not continue with the very same behavior that helped you, you will end up gaining all those pounds back and quitting.

Yet, this is what most people do. This behavior is dangerous because all the benefits you gained by losing weight and reducing your chances of having heart disease and diabetes have just been thrown away.

This behavior is similar to a driver who has learned how to drive defensively concluding after a minor fender-bender that defensive driving does not work. He or she then decides to go back to their old driving habits.

Who is more likely to get into a more serious accident on the road? The person who is driving defensively and paying attention to the rules of the road, or the person driving recklessly through traffic.

I think we all know who is likely to get into trouble. It is the same for maintaining your health. If you adopt some of the methods of healthy living that I have outlined in this book or that you have found from other sources, you will find yourself improving in all the parameters used to assess good health.

Naturally as these parameters like your BMI, blood pressure, cholesterol level, or more sleep per day improve, your risk for sudden death and unexpected illnesses like heart attack, and strokes will be highly reduced.

Notice that I did not say your chances of being ill will be eliminated. Just like defensive driving will not entirely eliminate your chances of having an accident, adopting a healthy living lifestyle will not make you completely immune to illness. However, nothing really beats that sense of feeling energetic and being ready for the day.

Once you start on the journey of healthy living, do not give up, even if you do not have the desired results at the beginning. Climbing the pyramid of healthy living is a step-by -step process.

TASK OF THE MOMENT.

*Keep your daily living ideas simple.

*Take a few ideas and use them consistently everyday.

*Do not let new ideas become distractions.

*Strive for daily consistency in your actions.

*Use every hour of the day for one healthy activity.

Create Your Own Blueprint for Healthy Living in 72 hours

Finally, you can put all that you have read and learned together to create your own individualized blueprint for transformative health within 72 hours.

Use the first 24 hours or first day to learn as much as you can about yourself. You can use part 1 of this book as your blueprint for transformative change. Do your health and cardiovascular risk assessment as described in the introduction and the first few chapters of this book. This assessment will give you an idea of your health status and your physical measurements and physiological measurements. Be sure to include your weight, height, waist circumference, blood pressure and pulse rate.

Using the measurements you have, calculate your BMI. This is a very good indicator of your overall health status.

The second step you need to do is to write down the patterns that are most prominent in your life during the past 72 hours. Identify and write down your:

*Eating pattern

*Working pattern

*Relationship pattern

*Activity pattern

*And Meditation pattern.

Write down your meals and snacks, how much TV you watch, and how you typically deal with your emotions like anger and sadness. Be accurate and specific.

In the second 24 hours or second day set up an appointment with your health care provider to enable you get a more detailed picture of your metabolic profile, especially your cholesterol level and other tests relevant to your family and medical history. See a nutritionist or dietitian for a more detailed nutritional analysis. If you are not able to do this, work with results from your first 24 hours of assessment.

In the third 24 hours or third day which will complete your 72 hour time frame begin to write down the components of your healthy living blueprint for the Long haul. Make this your own personalized list of actions and pledges that will help you transform your health and life. This basically means taking some detailed transformative actions and applying them to yourself and your circumstances.

Here is an example of a list you can make on the third day of your 72 hour time frame:

*Quit smoking now or plan to stop.

*Eat grains, vegetables, fruits, milk and beans, and use the right oils like cranola and olive oils.

*Eat at least 10g rams of fibers daily through eating cereals like oats and whole wheat bread.

*Eat at least five servings of fruits and vegetables daily.

*Eat a delicious red apple with every meal.

*Read your nutritional label before you buy or use your food products.

*Cut down your food portions by at least one-third.

*Eat your food in one location without TV.

*Eat fish and skinless poultry like chicken or turkey.

*Drink low-fat milk or eat low fat yoghurt.

*Walk at least 30 minutes everyday.

*Take a deep breath before you respond to stressful situations.

*Sleep at least six to eight hours a day.

*Cut down on unnecessary expenses.

*Call a friend today.

*Review your finances.

*Help at least one person each day.

*Meditate or say a prayer or do both.

*Form a healthy living-group of friends and family members.

*Write down your feelings and experiences.

*Repeat your blood pressure check.

*Weigh yourself regularly.

*Take your multivitamins regularly.

*Keep your appointment with your healthcare providers.

*Keep eating right even after a lapse.

*Do your yearly physical.

*Do your screening tests as recommended by your healthcare providers.

*Become familiar with your family and medical history.

*Review your health insurance regularly.

*Get more education.

*Protect your home from falls and accidents.

*Work for the future everyday.

*Continue to write down your emotions periodically.

*Forgive yourself and others daily.

*Keep quiet if you have nothing positive to say.

*Review and modify this list as it fits your individual needs and circumstances.

There you have it! These are the elements of the individualized 72 hour blueprint for healthy Living. You are welcome to use them and begin to transform your health immediately.

The key to success with **The Compass Health Transformer** is to keep things simple and to take action everyday. You do not need to wait to have all the components of your health assessment or even your comprehensive health review to begin your journey of healthy living. You can begin to take action with the knowledge you have, while you continue to learn more about yourself and your different **compass health profiles.**

www.ingramcontent.com/pod-product-compliance
Lightning Source LLC
Chambersburg,PA
CBHW070231290526
45789CB00004B/1572